Mindfulness Over Migraines

Mindfulness
Over Migraines

Stop Your Migraine in Minutes . . .
Naturally and Affordably

Cynthia Perkins, M.Ed.

Published by Cynthia A. Perkins, USA

© 2012 by Cynthia A. Perkins
Published in the United States of America

ISBN: 978-0-9841446-2-4

Cover Design by Andrew Perkins, www.andrewscustomwebdesign.com

Edited by Brenda Judy, www.publishersplanet.com

Bamboo Artwork by www.iStockphoto.com/chaluk

Disclaimer: The information in this book has not been evaluated by the Food and Drug Administration. The author is not a medical doctor, and any information in this book is not intended to diagnose, treat, cure or prevent any disease.

The information shared in this book is designed for educational purposes only, based on the personal and professional experiences and opinions of the author, and should not be taken as professional medical advice or used as a substitute for medical care or psychological counseling. With all medical or mental health conditions, you should consult a qualified medical or mental health professional before putting any of these suggestions to use.

You agree the author is not responsible for any adverse effects or consequences that may result, either directly or indirectly, from the suggestions contained herein and are aware that the author makes no guarantees on the outcome of recovery. Results and benefits may vary from person to person.

Mindfulness is best used for chronic pain, not acute pain. If you are experiencing acute pain of any kind, you should seek professional medical assistance immediately.

http://www.holistichelp.net

"Life's not about waiting for the storm to pass. It's about learning to dance in the rain."

~Vivian Green

Table of Contents

ONE

What is Mindfulness?

I had been practicing mindfulness for more than twenty years before realizing it, because I used different words to describe the process. As I wrote about managing chronic pain syndromes for a couple of decades, I used the words like go into the pain, embrace, become one with, accept, surrender, flow with the pain, experience it completely or let the pain flow through you.

As a woman who has dealt with a variety of painful conditions in my lifetime, including chronic migraines and headaches, myofacial pain, atypical trigeminal neuralgia, fibromyalgia, gallbladder issues, and irritable bowel—and one who is incapable of and unwilling to take prescription medications unless I'm dying—I had no choice but to find an alternative way of dealing with my pain.

Although our first instinct is to resist pain, I have learned through my personal experience that pain of all kinds—the physical, emotional and spiritual—are managed most effectively through acceptance. When we experience our pain in its entirety, it not only loses its power over us and reduces its ability to disrupt our life, but it enables us to live a richer and more fulfilling life. Then, to my surprise, I discovered that science actually backs this up and these are many of the same principles that are taught in mindfulness.

I've studied numerous psychological techniques, and healing and spiritual paths throughout my life, but I'm not the type of person who embraces labels, rigid definitions or dogma of any kind as I find it becomes confining, controlling and limiting.

Whether it's a spiritual practice, a psychological technique or a health strategy, I don't believe in making anyone or anything a god, and I don't like getting caught up in custom, worshipping the guru, tradition, formalities, etc. I like to boil things down to the bare bones, extract the basic premise and then do my own thing with it. I encourage you to do the same. I find when we get too focused on the technique, mentor or guru, tradition, etc., then what we are trying to achieve becomes much more difficult to attain and the "real" experience gets lost.

So, I typically avoid aligning myself too stringently with any particular philosophy. However, over the years, as I've been trying to teach people my approach for alleviating and managing chronic pain and living a fuller, more meaningful life, it was difficult to put a name on the process. I find mindfulness to be very useful in describing the work that I do without feeling controlled by rigid principles; thus, I have embraced the word and the concept.

This change came about when I watched a webinar by Dr. Charles Gant on the topic of mindfulness, and I was like, "Hey, I've been practicing that for years, but that's not what I called it." Also during all those years, I had been using mindfulness to get me "through" the migraine. In this webinar I learned that mindfulness could be used to "stop" the migraine.[1] I then did some research and discovered that mindfulness is being used for pain syndromes of all kinds quite successfully.

For example, in a study by Jon Kabat-Zinn and others, individuals with chronic migraine, tension headaches, as well as backache were able to significantly reduce their pain, as well as other symptoms that often accompany pain like anxiety and depression and loss of functionality, with mindfulness-based meditation.[2]

In another study by Jon Kabat-Zinn, M.D., at the Stress Reduction Clinic at the University of Massachusetts, participants were able to reduce chronic pain by more than 50 percent. The participants in this study also experienced an increased ability to perform their daily activities and long-term improvements in mood.[3]

Patients with Irritable Bowel Syndrome (IBS) were able to reduce symptoms by 38 percent, and also experienced significant reduction in psychological distress and improvement in quality of life, with regular practice of mindfulness in a study performed at the University of North Carolina at Chapel Hill.[4]

In another study of migraineurs and meditation, 72 percent of the participants experienced fewer migraines, developed a higher pain tolerance, less anxiety, and a higher level of headache related self-efficacy and overall sense of well-being.[5]

At the Wake Forest and Marquette University study, subjects with migraines were able to reduce pain intensity by 57 percent and perception of pain by 40 percent, which was also illustrated by brain changes in an MRI.[6]

Mindfulness meditation is proving to be of significant help in not only reducing migraines or chronic pain, but improvements in mood, outlook on life and illness, increased coping skills, enhanced sense of well-being, changes in perception of pain, higher tolerance of pain, enhanced immune function, less fatigue and stress, and better sleep associated with cancer, fibromyalgia, arthritis, irritable bowel syndrome and more.

Numerous studies abound that find mindfulness meditation to be beneficial for improving a variety of conditions besides chronic pain, including high blood pressure, stress, heart disease, insomnia, depression, anxiety, drug and alcohol addiction, even AIDS and emotional pain of all kinds.

Although it was once considered an alternative treatment method, meditation is now not only acceptable but encouraged by a variety of physicians, hospitals and health care centers, in both the conventional and alternative medicine fields.

So, with a little experimentation, I learned with just a bit of tweaking to the technique I had been practicing for many years I could turn off the migraine completely, before it progressed. I also discovered that there is a specific manner, process and timing that must be applied to the mindfulness practice in order to alleviate migraine pain most effectively. That is what I am going to share with you in this book.

Before we get into the specific technique of relieving pain, let's first get an understanding of exactly what mindfulness is, why it is effective, and how we can apply it to migraines and other chronic pain syndromes of all kinds.

Jon Kabat-Zinn, the founder of the Mindfulness-Based Stress Reduction program at the University of Massachusetts Medical Center and considered to be the world's leading expert on mindfulness, describes mindfulness as, "Mindfulness means paying attention in a particular way; on purpose, in the present moment, and non-judgmentally."[7]

To expand further, mindfulness is the act of being more aware and conscious of the present moment, without judgment. Or, in other words, making a conscious choice to be aware and experience the present moment to the fullest without judgment, in all your activities, without dwelling in the past or the future. Other ways of thinking about it include…

> Experiencing that present moment, or your life, to the fullest and completely; regardless of whether that moment is positive or negative, painful or pleasurable, happy or sad. Feel and experience your feelings and sensations completely.
>
> Being completely aware and present.
>
> Focused on the experience of the moment, which is commonly referred to as living in the NOW.
>
> Quieting the noise. Noise is anything that interrupts the experience of the moment. (Internal chatter, thoughts, emotions or external noise like sounds, etc.)

Extracting yourself from your thoughts.

Conscious awareness and focused attention.

Recognizing that our thoughts are not necessarily reality, just thoughts that can be observed rather than producing a reaction.

Most people go through life mindlessly—disconnected, unaware and not paying attention—and miss out on the depth that life has to offer. Mindfulness is the opposite of mindless.

I find that thinking of mindfulness in the following way simplifies the concept: approaching all your experiences in life as if you are engaging in a passionate lovemaking session with the love of your life for the first time. Here is an example to help clarify further.

Mindfulness Example

One of the simplest ways to put mindfulness into practice and understand the concept is through food.

- When you eat, be one with your food as if you are in a deep meditation.

- Put your focus solely on your food and the experience of eating; tuning everything else out.

- Experience the sensation of the food on your tongue, the flavor and the sound of chewing completely.
- Be aware of each bite—the flavor, the smell, the texture and temperature in your mouth.
- Be "with" your food.
- Don't gobble things down mindlessly.
- Savor your food as if you are engaging in a long, slow, tender and passionate lovemaking session.
- Look at it, feel it, smell it and taste it completely.

Being more mindful of your food and the experience of eating enhances your health physically, emotionally and spiritually. Your food and your eating experience are much more flavorful, satisfying and fulfilling, all of which enhance mood and feelings of well-being. It allows time for your hunger hormones to communicate with your body, telling it when to stop eating; thus, it reduces cravings for carbs and you are less likely to overeat. Digestion is enhanced, which ensures delivery of more nutrients to the body and mind, and smoother transit throughout the gastrointestinal tract.

Although mindfulness has its roots in Buddhism and Eastern philosophy, and is often a considered a spiritual practice, the basic principles themselves are not attached to any particular religious element and can be used within the context of any belief system.

The goal in using mindfulness to alleviate migraines or chronic pain is not about the pursuit of spirituality, but enhanced spiritual health is an inherent quality of mindfulness, and this will be of great benefit as well. In my own exploration of chronic pain, and in my professional experience, I have found there are several intertwined levels of pain: the physical level, the emotional/psychological and the spiritual level. Where you find one, you typically find the other.

There is no area of your life that goes unscathed when you live with chronic migraines or a chronic pain condition. It affects us on all levels: the physical, emotional and spiritual, as well as cognitively and socially.

Severe physical pain (the physical level) is likely to cause emotional distress (the emotional level) as one struggles to cope with feelings of loss, grief and anger associated with diminished abilities or changes in lifestyle or identity. In forming a new identity that includes living with migraines or chronic pain, one may struggle with the spiritual pain (the spiritual level) of existential aloneness. Questions such as "Why me?" and "What is the purpose of my life now?" may arise.

The greatest beauty of mindfulness meditation is that it addresses each of these aspects equally; thus, the benefits you will acquire go well beyond relieving physical pain. Its ability to improve our emotional health and quality of life is a built-in positive side effect of the technique.

The practice of mindfulness-based meditation is one of the most powerful holistic self-care tools you can use to optimize your physical, mental and spiritual health. It's a simple and convenient technique that doesn't require any special skills or training. You will know how to do it adequately and put it to use by the time you finish reading this book.

TWO

The Science of
Mindfulness & Migraines

The science behind mindfulness tells us amazing things about the brain. Numerous studies have demonstrated that mindfulness meditation changes areas of the brain that are associated with memory, sense of self, empathy, compassion, introspection, anxiety, stress and fear.

Using neuroimagery on the brain, it has been found that mindfulness stimulates the frontal lobes of the brain, which increases our stress reducing neurotransmitters like dopamine, serotonin, GABA, endorphins and enkephalins, and reduces our primary stress inducing neurotransmitter, norepinephrine, that sets off the stress response system.

In *Zen and the Brain*, Dr. James Austin, a neurophysiologist at the University of Colorado, explains that meditation actually rewires the circuits in the brain. His theories have been confirmed with the latest brain imaging techniques.

Dr. Herbert Benson—a researcher who pioneered the health benefits of meditation and who's now at the Mind-Body Medical Institute, a facility that's associated with Harvard University and several Boston hospitals—tells us that meditation produces real physical changes that are biochemical in nature.[1]

When you meditate, you're generating alpha and/or theta brainwaves and, when you're generating alpha and theta brainwaves, it stimulates neurotransmitters in the brain that improve mood, decrease pain, slow the heart rate, incite relaxation and feelings of euphoria, and boosts the immune system. This is one of the primary reasons we reap so many health benefits from meditation. Alpha and theta waves are both associated with high levels of creativity, intuition and insight; so, during those states of mind, you get the added benefit of being more creative, intuitive and insightful.

As soon as you close your eyes, even when you're awake and not meditating, your brain slows down to the alpha cycle. Alpha brainwaves are associated with being in a relaxed, non-aroused state of mind. This is why closing your eyes throughout the day instantly helps you feel more relaxed—you're slowing down your brainwaves.

Theta waves are associated with deeper levels of meditation, daydreaming, intuition, the subconscious mind, spiritual experiences, periods of insight, dreaming while sleeping, and high levels of creativity. They, too, may produce feelings of euphoria, which are more intense than those experienced in alpha. Not only that, theta waves are believed to boost the immune system as well. Theta waves are experienced by most people in the seconds right before they fall asleep.

Neurons in the brain are "wired" to produce neurotransmitters like serotonin, dopamine, GABA and beta-endorphins at certain brain wave frequencies.[2] Neurotransmitters are responsible for a vast number of functions throughout the mind and body, and regulating pain perception and mood states are two of the most important, as well as our sleep cycle and stress response system. They increase empathy, compassion, introspection, self-awareness, inner peace, relaxation, happiness, joy and pleasure, and reduce pain, fear, anger, anxiety and stress. Other studies have found that mindfulness meditation stimulates melatonin, our primary sleep hormone, as well as boosts our immune system.

Dopamine is the primary neurotransmitter that regulates our pleasure or reward pathway and aids in the regulation of emotional responses and motor function. It also helps with brain focus, attention and energy. When there isn't sufficient dopamine, you lack motivation, pleasure in life, ability to pay to attention and remain focused, and this often leads to addiction.

Serotonin is also responsible for regulating emotions and provides us with feelings of happiness, a sense of well-being, self-esteem, serenity and relaxation. It's our natural antidepressant. Insufficient levels of serotonin are associated with depression, anxiety and addiction.

GABA is our primary inhibitory neurotransmitter and produces a calming and relaxing effect on the body and mind. It's our natural sedative like Xanax, alcohol or Valium. A lack of GABA may cause anxiety, obsessive compulsive disorders or addiction.

Endorphins and enkephalins are naturally occurring opiate-like neurotransmitters in the brain, and their primary role is to relieve or reduce pain. However, they also produce euphoria, a sense of well-being, improved self-esteem, relaxation and influence mood. They may also boost the immune system and slow down the growth of cancer cells.

Beta-endorphins are believed to be significantly more potent than morphine. Think of them as your body's natural painkiller. For example, if you hit your thumb with the hammer or shut your fingers in the car door, beta-endorphins are released to deal with the pain.

Therefore, by stimulating your endorphins, you can produce your own opiates that relieve migraines, headaches, backaches or any kind of pain you're dealing with.

The Autonomic Nervous System

One of the most important roles our neurotransmitters play is modulating the autonomic nervous system. The autonomic nervous system, also known as the involuntary nervous system, regulates those facets in the body that occur automatically, such as breathing, blood pressure, digestion, heartbeat, bladder function, and narrowing or widening of the blood vessels. It is composed of two branches—the parasympathetic nervous system and the sympathetic nervous system.

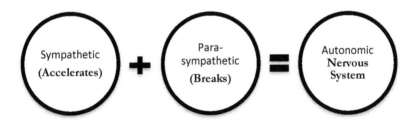

Sympathetic

The sympathetic nervous system is also known as our stress response system, or the fight or flight system, and is set into motion when we experience stress. It increases our heart rate and blood pressure, dilates pupils, restricts circulation, slows down digestion, relaxes the bladder, enhances our senses, makes us more alert and aware, and provides a boost in energy so that we are capable of dealing with the stressful situation effectively. It increases energy and is often referred to as the accelerator of the autonomic nervous system.

Parasympathetic

The job of the parasympathetic nervous system is the exact opposite. Once the stressful event is over, it brings the heart rate and blood pressure back to normal, constricts pupils, improves circulation, enhances digestion, calms us down, brings senses back to normal, contracts the bladder, and puts us into a state of rest and relaxation. It conserves energy and is often referred to as the breaks of the autonomic nervous system.

The sympathetic nervous system is triggered into action in an area of the brain known as the locus ceruleus any time we experience stress of any kind. Stress comes in many different forms, which may include emotional stress, oxidative stress, toxic stress, infectious stress, sensory stress, endocrine stress, spiritual stress, energetic stress, structural stress and more.

The locus ceruleus resides in the brain stem and it then releases norepinephrine, which is an excitatory neurotransmitter that sets off the fight or flight response. It only takes one neuron in the locus ceruleus to instantly ignite all the cells in the body because, when we are faced with a threat, there is no time for delay.

This triggers the amygdala, which is connected to emotions like fear and anger that we often experience when under stress, and the hypothalamus. The hypothalamus then stimulates the pituitary to release Adrenocorticotropic Hormone (ACTH), which then stimulates the adrenal glands to release cortisol, and preganglion sympathetic neurons stimulate the adrenal medulla to release epinephrine.

This system is called the fight or flight system, also known as the stress response system or the sympathetic nervous system, and takes place in the area of the brain called the limbic system. It is designed to protect us from threats like predators. It is a survival mechanism. In our earlier development as a species, it protected us from predators like lions. We would see the lion and the stress response system would go into action to help us deal with the stress of escaping the lion.

We would escape the lion, the sympathetic nervous system would turn off and the body would return to its pre-stress state called the parasympathetic state, which is a state of rest, digest and relaxation. The lions we face today come in many different forms, like financial instability, environmental toxins, relationship conflict, loss of employment, poor diet and nutrition, neurotransmitter and hormone imbalances, overgrowth of unfriendly organisms in the Gastrointestinal Tract (GI) tract, and more.

When the autonomic nervous system is functioning as it should, the sympathetic nervous system and the parasympathetic nervous system work in perfect harmony together to maintain balance in the body. The sympathetic nervous system provides us with the tools we need to respond to stress adequately, and the parasympathetic nervous system restores us to our normal state of peace and tranquility.

The problem in this day and age is that we are surrounded by lions (stress) everywhere we go and we can't escape them, so we are thrust into the sympathetic state on a frequent basis and this is taking a toll on our physical, emotional and spiritual health.

Dysautonomia, or autonomic nervous system dysfunction, occurs when these two systems fail to work together in harmony. The most common scenario is the sympathetic nervous system remains dominant most of the time and the parasympathetic rarely turns on.

When this occurs, the body remains in a state of fight or flight at all times. The stress response system never turns off. If the body remains in a state of fight or flight at all times, then many degenerative processes begin to happen and result in a variety of chronic health conditions and overall poor health because it is only supposed to be used for brief emergencies.

The stress response system was designed to deal with brief emergencies that threaten survival. It isn't supposed to last very long because the body cannot sustain itself for very long in this state. The natural and preferred state of the mind and body is the parasympathetic state, because it is regenerative. However, it is willing to forgo its preferred parasympathetic state to deal with acute emergencies and will remain in that state if the emergency continues.

If the brain and the body remain in the sympathetic fight or flight state for too long and too often, it is degenerative; it breaks us down. If this cycle continues, then eventually the system burns out. This cycle results in dysautonomia or autonomic nervous system dysfunction.

Dysfunction in the autonomic nervous system is a primary contributing factor to migraines, headaches and chronic pain syndromes of all kinds, including conditions like fibromyalgia, myofacial pain, irritable bowel, back pain and Multiple Sclerosis (MS), as well as other conditions like insomnia, anxiety disorders, depression, adrenal fatigue, addiction, high blood pressure, heart disease, impotency, circulation disorders, violent behaviors, autism, gastrointestinal disorder, Gulf War Syndrome (GWS), chemical sensitivity and many more.

When the sympathetic fight or flight system is activated for any reason, be it toxins or emotional stress, the frontal lobes of the brain are triggered as well to cope with the stressful event. Serotonin, dopamine, GABA, endorphins/enkephalins, etc., are released to inhibit the locus ceruleus, amygdala, thalamus and hypothalamus to balance the fight or flight system. If the frontal lobes aren't working properly, then fight or flight cannot be regulated sufficiently. You stay in fight or flight all the time.

Serotonin, dopamine, GABA, endorphins/enkephalins, endocannabinoids, taurine and histamine are neurotransmitters that all oppose norepinephrine; thus, they turn off the sympathetic fight or flight system. They are released during times of stress to bring us back to the parasympathetic state. Since we are all in a state of chronic stress on a frequent basis, our levels of neurotransmitters are frequently drained and they aren't available in sufficient numbers to deal with the stress at hand.

Therefore, when you engage in mindfulness meditation, you are stimulating an abundance of these neurotransmitters that will modulate your stress response system and return you to the preferred and regenerative parasympathetic state.

Our frontal lobes are connected to all the other parts of the cerebral cortex, like our intellect, and can inhibit those areas when it's activated; thus, turning off the constant stream of thoughts. Additionally, it is also connected to the thalamus, our command center for sensation. The fontal lobes influence the part of the thalamus that gaits what sensations are allowed into the brain. So, this means that the frontal lobes are involved in the gaiting process.

For example, the thalamus tells you to pay attention to an intense pain in your back, but the frontal lobes can override this message when it's activated and take your attention away from the pain. This is one of the mechanisms that enable mindfulness to be such an effective method of pain relief. Therefore, it appears that the ability to use our breath or any focal point as a gaiting process to inhibit intrusive thoughts (or any noise) is hardwired into our brain.

Because the frontal lobes are connected to all other parts of the cerebral cortex, including our intellect and the thalamus, it can override the constant internal chatter and is involved in the gaiting process of sensory information.[3]

Basically, what all this means is that mindfulness turns off the sympathetic nervous system and boosts neurotransmitters.

Although the exact science of why a migraine occurs is not fully understood at this time, what we do know for sure is that it is a complex condition involving a variety of overlapping factors like the brain stem, neurons and neurotransmitters, the vascular system and blood vessels, hormones, the trigeminal nerve, and the autonomic nervous system.

The predominant theory for many years in regard to the underlying cause of migraines was that it was primarily a vascular condition. However, more recent studies challenge this theory and suggest that it is the autonomic nervous system that is at the seat of the problem, with the swelling of blood vessels and other aspects being secondary, as each of them are interconnected to one another and the autonomic nervous system. Studies have also found that not everyone who gets a migraine has swelling of blood vessels.

As we see in our discussion throughout this book, mindfulness has a direct impact on each of these contributing factors since it targets the brain and the autonomic nervous system. This is why it is so effective for relieving migraines or chronic pain of all kinds. Although pain is experienced in many different areas of the body, pain of any kind is regulated in the brain and influenced by the autonomic nervous system.

The crucial point you want to be aware of in regard to the autonomic nervous system is that it becomes dysfunctional for a variety of contributing factors, which may include, but is not limited to:

- emotional trauma, such as childhood abuse, war, poverty, violence, surviving a natural disaster, loss of a loved one or any form of great loss
- environmental toxins
- poor diet
- sugar
- overconsumption of starchy carbs
- caffeine
- nicotine
- drugs and alcohol
- nutritional deficiencies

- metabolic problems like hypoglycemia

- excessive oxidative stress

- hormone and neurotransmitter imbalances

- chronic emotional stress

- structural disorders like Temporomandibular joint disorders (TMJ)

- food sensitivities

- overgrowth of unfriendly organisms like candida yeast, parasites and bacteria

- physical trauma like a sports injury, a car accident or tooth extraction

- chronic stress of any kind

- lack of meaning and purpose in your life

Thus, why there are so many varying types of triggers for people with migraines or underlying contributors to chronic pain of other kinds. Addressing these underlying factors is also important for restoring balance to the autonomic nervous system, and alleviating your migraines or chronic pain.

Afferent and Efferent Neurons

When using mindfulness to relieve a migraine or chronic pain, the source of your chronic pain will be used as the focal point of your meditation. You'll learn the exact technique in chapter six but, for now, you just need to learn the whys and whats.

Mindfulness can be as effective, if not more so, at alleviating migraines or other chronic pain as prescription drugs. By using the source of the chronic pain as the focal point of your mindfulness exercise, pain can dissolve and dissipate completely.

It's important to note that there is a very distinct difference between being preoccupied with your pain and being mindful of your pain. Being preoccupied will increase the pain level, while being mindful will reduce it. In the mindfulness webinar presented by Dr. Charles Gant, he described it like this.

We have two types of neurons, efferent and afferent. Efferent (motor/autonomic) neurons carry information from the central computer (our brain) back to the body, while afferent (sensory neurons) carry information from the body (head, gallbladder, back, heart, muscles, GI tract, etc.) back to the brain.

The secret to relieving the pain is to move your focus away from the motor pathways (efferent) and open up your sensory pathways (afferent). This allows the body to communicate with the brain and guide it to the area where the attention is needed.

So, when you zero in on the location of the pain, as you'll learn how to do farther ahead, then you are essentially telling the brain, "Here is the problem, right here." The brain can then go to work on the problem. All your neurons can go to work on the area of the pain and everything else is tuned out.

At any given time, there may be a few million neurons directed at the pain you're experiencing; however, when you bring your full awareness to the pain, and experience it in its entirety, you bring it to the attention of your frontal lobes. When the frontal lobes become involved, then you have 5 or 10 billion neurons that become attached to the pain and go to work on it.

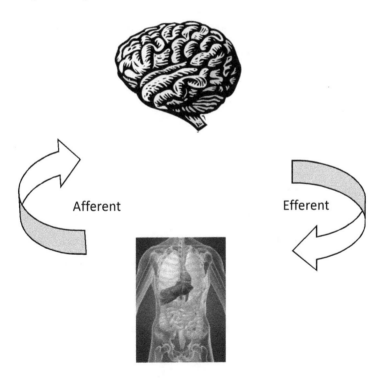

This opens up the afferent/efferent pathways and provides an abundance of afferent information to be pipelined directly to the brain; telling the command control center exactly where the problem resides. The brain didn't have anything to work with before, so it didn't know what to do with the pain; but, when you hand it all this information, it knows how to correct the problem.

It's like the brain says, "Ah, I see . . . the problem is right here. Let me get to work on that."

Pain relieving drugs, or even natural herbs, disrupt this process. They deaden the sensory pathway (afferent pathway), and impair communication between the efferent and afferent neurons. Thus, there is no way to ever get well—instead of healing, addiction happens because you have cut the central computer out of the healing process.

Pain relieving drugs and herbs temporarily boost your neurotransmitters and turn off your sympathetic nervous system by mimicking your natural neurotransmitters, which temporarily alleviates symptoms; thereby, tricking you into believing they are making you better. However, because the boost is artificial and too intense, the brain responds by making less neurotransmitters because it thinks it has enough.

Remember, neurotransmitters are needed to modulate the autonomic nervous system. When they aren't present, they can't counteract norepinephrine and turn off your sympathetic nervous system. Without these neurotransmitters, we cannot turn off fight or flight. Additionally, they modulate pain. If they aren't present to do this job, then pain increases or runs amuck.

When this happens, a vicious cycle ensues: neurotransmitter levels drop lower, then you become dependent on the drug or herbs to bring them back up. The more you turn to the substance, the more your neurotransmitters become depleted and the more dominant your sympathetic nervous system becomes. More and more symptoms develop, and mental and physical health continues to decline. Psychotropic drugs or herbs become a way of anesthetizing the autonomic nervous system.

Addicts of all kinds are unconsciously trying to restore balance to their brain chemistry, soothe their autonomic nervous system and find inner peace by using psychotropic chemicals to artificially stimulate their neurotransmitters.

The drugs or herbs must be removed in order to return to the parasympathetic state. There cannot be improvement in psychiatric or physiological health if one remains dependent on psychotropics. Psychotropic drugs and herbs take the brain, which is the captain of the ship for the autonomic nervous system, out of the ball game. The brain needs to get communication from the body so it knows what to do.

The afferent and efferent neurons take information to and from the frontal lobe to other areas of the brain, like the cerebral cortex, limbic system, thalamus, visual cortex, temporal lobes and somatosensory cortex. Thus, a feed-forward/feedback loop exists that connects the emotional brain, the survival brain and the frontal lobes.

Allowing someone to experience their pain is a foreign concept to most of the medical establishment and, consequently, society in general. Instead, they encourage everyone to anesthetize and avoid their pain, which makes it difficult for those experiencing pain to grasp the concept I am presenting here and understand that feeling their pain is the true road to relief.

When you have a willingness to embrace your pain, let it exist and sit with it, you give your brain the information it needs to take care of the problem.

Most chronic pain disorders respond favorably to mindfulness, but I have found it be exceptionally beneficial for migraines, headaches, myofacial pain, TMJ, tension headaches, arthritic type pain, fibro-myalgia, irritable bowel, generalized muscle aches, atypical trigeminal neuralgia, backaches and even gallbladder pain.

THREE

Breathing Fundamentals

Although breathwork or deep breathing exercises can be very beneficial as a stand-alone practice, they typically go hand in hand with meditation. It's hard to talk about meditating without talking about breath, because they are interconnected. It's important that you know how to breathe properly before learning the mindfulness technique for migraines because you will be using it extensively.

Like meditation, deep breathing produces soothing, relaxing and pleasure-inducing alpha brainwaves; calms the excitatory neurotransmitters; stimulates melatonin and turns off the stress response system;

and, thus, relieves anxiety and stress instantly, and promotes better sleep.

As you learned in the previous chapter, alpha brainwaves also stimulate dopamine, serotonin and beta-endorphins, the body's built-in natural pain reliever, and stimulate creativity as well. Therefore, when you combine breathwork with your meditation technique, you double all your benefits.

In *Breathing: The Master Key to Self Healing*, Dr. Andrew Weil tells us that breathing is the only function in the human body that is done either completely unconsciously or completely consciously. It can be a voluntary or involuntary act, and it is governed by two distinct sets of muscles and nerves depending on which mode is in use—the involuntary nerves and muscles or the voluntary.

Each set of muscles and nerves can fully drive and manage the system. Therefore, the breath has this phenomenal, unique characteristic that enables it to affect the involuntary nervous system. It is the only function in the human body that has this ability. We can use our voluntary breathing to influence our involuntary nervous system, also known as the autonomic nervous system.

This is where the importance of breath comes into play. Voluntary acts of breathing with specific techniques can be used to turn off the sympathetic nervous system and turn on the parasympathetic nervous system. When the sympathetic nervous system is dominant, the breathing is fast, short and shallow. When the parasympathetic nervous system is activated, we breathe slower, deeper and longer. Therefore, if we intentionally breathe slower, deeper and longer, we can turn on the parasympathetic nervous system. We can calm down, rev up or harmonize the nervous system with our breath.

As we discussed previously, over activity of the sympathetic nervous system is believed to be the major contributor to migraines, chronic pain of all kinds, as well as a whole host of other health conditions such as anxiety disorders, depression, heart disease, high blood pressure, insomnia, gastrointestinal disorders, adrenal disorders, hyperactivity, multiple chemical sensitivity, addiction, autism, ulcers, obesity and many more. So, restoring balance to the autonomic nervous system is a crucial component for optimizing health for everyone.

Our goal in breathwork is to change our breathing qualities. When we are under stress, upset, angry or afraid, our breath is shallow, irregular, noisy and rapid. In a relaxed state, our breath is quiet, slow, deep and long. Therefore, we want to focus on making our breath deeper, longer, quieter, regular and slower as often as possible. The more often we do this, the more often we put the parasympathetic nervous system in the driver seat and calm down the sympathetic nervous system.

How to Breathe Properly

1. When you inhale, your abdomen should protrude, not your chest. When you exhale, your abdomen should flatten.

2. As you breathe in, you should breathe in slowly through the nose, not the mouth, until the lungs are almost full. When you exhale, it should be slow and controlled until almost all air is expelled.

3. Each breath should be through the nose—deep, complete, long, slow and controlled.

4. Place your hands on your abdomen. If they rise and fall with each breath, then you are breathing correctly.

Use your breath as needed throughout your day during times of high anxiety, stress or disharmony. Wherever you are, just stop and take a few minutes to close your eyes and take several deep breaths using the proper breathing procedure described above.

Basic Deep Breathing Exercise

Here is the breathing exercise I have found to be most beneficial, practiced with mindfulness or independently.

1. Open your mouth and exhale.

2. Close your mouth and take a long slow breath in through the nostrils as described above in "How to Breathe Properly."

3. Keep your mouth closed and breathe out through the nose—long, slow and controlled—as described above. You'll notice that immediately your heart rate slows down and you probably feel more relaxed and less stressful.

4. Each time you breathe in and out, that is considered a round. So, do at least four or five rounds; you can go up to fifteen or twenty if you can or need to. You can stop once you begin to feel the relaxation radiate through your body and mind, or continue with a few more rounds for deeper relaxation.

5. Close your eyes, if possible. Closing your eyes enhances the benefits of your breath, because this immediately activates alpha brainwaves and incites relaxation. Keep this point in mind, because closing the eyes periodically throughout the day is another great way to relieve stress by itself. However, if it isn't possible to close your eyes, the breathing alone will work as well.

The way that you breathe is crucial. The mouth must be shut, the breath must come in and out through the nose, and you must breathe from the abdomen. You must not inhale or exhale too deeply, breathe too shallow or fast, or hold the breath very long, or it can trigger the sympathetic nervous system. Don't hold the breath in the body. You want the breath to flow through the body and out.

The position of the eyes is also important. I have found if you put pressure on your eyes by looking too far in one direction, it can trigger the sympathetic nervous system as well. The eyes should be closed; but don't close too tightly, don't roll them around in your head, don't look upwards or sideways, and don't put any strain on them. Just look straight ahead without pressure, as if you are looking through a hole in the middle of your forehead. If you practice with your eyes open, the same guidelines apply.

Your body and mind may resist at first, so be gentle. You may have to train your body and mind by easing them into the practice a little at a time. Go slow at first and engage only for a few minutes. Over time you'll begin to feel the positive effects and then your mind will get more responsive and willing, and a snowball effect will occur. The more you practice, the more effective it becomes; and, the more effective it becomes, the more responsive you are.

In *Breathing: The Master Key to Self Healing*, Dr. Andrew Weil tells us that if we practice this type of breathing on a regular basis, then eventually we can train the breath to follow this pattern on its own and the nervous system will respond accordingly. Repetition and frequency are important. With the continuous repetition of deep, slow, long, quiet breaths, we can restore balance between the sympathetic and parasympathetic nervous system. We feel more harmonious in body, mind and spirit; the nervous system and organs function more smoothly.

When you breathe through your nose, as described above, you can use your breath to not only relieve migraines or other chronic pain, but you can also boost energy; clarify and quiet the mind; relieve tension and stress; lesson the intensity of symptoms of any health conditions you have; improve sleep; relax, calm and soothe the body and mind; quiet the deeper or core self; and help you be more spiritually connected. You will also oxygenate your body, help your body to detoxify better and boost the immune system.

Sometimes I can turn off a migraine or some other type of pain with deep breathing alone, but it depends on the trigger and intensity. Just repeat the basic deep breathing exercise for 5 to 15 minutes. You can use a little a trial and error to see how it works for you, but it's important to master the basic breathing steps above, because they are an integral component of the mindfulness over migraine core technique that you are about to learn.

FOUR

Understanding the Basics of Mindfulness Meditation

Before we apply mindfulness meditation to alleviating our migraines or chronic pain, we first want to gain an understanding of the basic process.

The simplest and most basic mindfulness meditation practice uses the breath for the focal point (or anchor) of the meditation. This is the easiest way to learn, and once the basic principle is mastered, then you can carry it over to many other focal points like pain.

The goal in mindfulness meditation is to quiet the noise. The noise is anything around you that disrupts the meditation process. There is inner noise, like thoughts and the inner commentator; and outside noise, like people, sounds, etc. As you become more skilled with mindfulness, you can learn how to make the noise become a focal point, but for now we'll focus on the breath.

Lie down, or sit down.

Close your eyes.

Take a deep breath in through your nose, with your mouth closed.

Breathe from your abdomen, not your chest.

Let your breath out through the nose in a slow and controlled manner (as you learned in the previous chapter). Repeat several times.

During this process you stay focused on the breath and the process of breathing.

Follow the breath in and out. To use the words of Dr. Charles Gant, "Feel the feeling, sense the sensation, moment to moment."[1]

If thoughts intrude, which they ultimately will, then just acknowledge them and release them without judgment. As Jon Kabat-Zinn, says, "This is what minds do."[2] Gently and persistently bring the mind back to the breath.

Just breathe and focus.

Optional

You can place your hand on your abdomen to help anchor your focus more if needed. Then you can focus on the rise and fall of your hand as you breathe in and out.

If additional help is needed to stay focused, you can say quietly in your mind each time you breathe in and breathe out, "In" and "Out." This uses your intellect to keep thoughts from intruding in the process.

In the depths of mindfulness, there is no distinction between the breather and the breath, the feeler and the feeling, the experiencer and the experience—they are one in the same.

As we discussed in the "Breathing Fundamentals" chapter, deep breathing exercises have a variety of benefits physically, emotionally and spiritually as well, so using the breath as the focal point in the manner I have described doubles the physical, emotional and spiritual benefits that can be attained. Even when I use a different focal point, I usually like to combine it with the breath.

Mindfulness Every Day

So, that's the basics of mindfulness meditation. Once you master this technique, then you can apply it to a variety of other focal points or anchors. For example, you could use music, the sound of rain or crickets, silence, a tree, or a body part. One of my favorite mindfulness exercises uses the hand as the focal point.

One of the aspects I love the most about mindfulness meditation is that all the benefits can be achieved in a few short minutes; you don't have to find long periods of time in your day to sit down for a formal and disciplined meditation session. Just a few minutes here and there suffice just fine and produce instant relaxation, inner peace, reduced stress, better mood and decreased pain.

However, keep in mind that meditation is only one method to attain mindfulness. There are many other ways it can be achieved throughout your daily life activities, such as gardening, baking, walking, exercising and even making love. By simply becoming aware and focused on the experience of the moment—whatever the moment may be—and quieting your inner commentator, mindfulness can be reached. As you learn how to put it into practice in your day-to-day life on a regular basis, life becomes a meditation.

FIVE

When to do Mindfulness
for Migraines
(Timing is Crucial for Success)

If you live with chronic migraines or have them periodically, you are probably aware that most migraines have a cycle that they go through. At first you get a few little signs that a migraine may be coming; this may vary somewhat from person to person. Some people get auras, but not everyone. I have never experienced an aura, but I have numerous early warning signs.

There are many signals that alert you of the on-coming danger before the skull-splitting pain arrives. There may be visual disturbances, heart palpitations, increased blood pressure or pulse rate, irritability, heightened sensitivity to sound or smell, and little twinges of pain. Then the pain slowly builds up and grows more intense over a period of time. After the pain rises to a certain degree, there is a peak. At the peak, the pain is at its highest level. After the peak, it feels like there is a break in the storm and the pain level starts to decline slowly. Eventually, the pain is gone and you are back to baseline.

The time frame that this cycle occurs varies from person to person, and may even vary within the same person from migraine to migraine. One person may go through their cycle in 4 hours, while another may go through their cycle in 10 hours, and yet another may go through their cycle in 24 hours, etc. For example, most of my migraines last for 16 hours before the peak breaks; however, every now and then I get one that lasts 6 hours, 10 hours, 24 hours or some other odd number.

The key to using mindfulness effectively for migraines is to use it at the very first signs that a migraine is going to occur—before the pain begins to build. This is crucial.

The sooner you start the mindfulness practice, the more successful you will be in alleviating the pain. Once the pain cycle hits a certain point in the building process, then there is no stopping it. It is like a runaway train at that point. I call this the "point of no return." See the bell-shape curve below to clarify further.

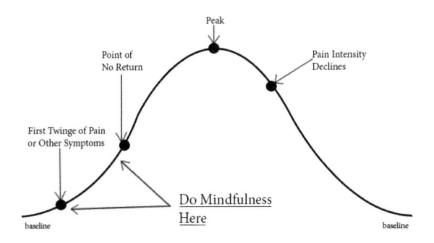

It's interesting to note that most prescription medications for migraines have the same criteria—the medication is most effective when used within 15 to 20 minutes of the first signs of a migraine. So, this seems to be a universal aspect for derailing migraines.

Most of the studies I've mentioned in this book say that about 30 percent to 70 percent of the subjects are successful, and the subjects experienced about 50 percent to 70 percent improvement. Using the technique you're about to learn, I have refined my skills to the point that I have about an 80 percent success rate for <u>completely</u> turning off the migraines that occur when I'm not sleeping. I have chronic migraines, which, in my case, means I can experience anywhere from three to twenty a month. It varies month to month, but I'm derailing a lot of migraines.

Now, those that occur when I'm sleeping are a different story. As we discussed above, in the bell-shape curve, we must get to the practice before the migraine progresses to "the point of no return." When I'm sleeping I'm not able to intervene, unless I have woken up to go to the bathroom and discover that a migraine has snuck in like a thief in the night. If I wake before it hits "the point of no return," then all is good and I can put a stop to it, but sometimes I wake when it is already too late.

Once in a great while, I may get a migraine that comes sweeping in so quickly and intensely while I'm awake that there is not time to do the practice, because I'm immediately at "the point of no return." You may have this experience as well from time to time, but most migraines do not follow this pattern.

The key point you want to take away here is that you must do the mindfulness practice as soon as you feel that first little twinge of pain. Immediately! The longer you wait, the less effective it becomes.

If I do the mindfulness practice within the first minute or two of the first signs of pain, it typically dissolves almost instantly. If it's 5 or 10 minutes after the pain arrives, then it takes 5 or 10 minutes to dissolve. If its 10 or 15 minutes before doing my practice, it takes about 15, or maybe 30, minutes to dissolve. If it's after 20 to 30 minutes, then it usually stops being effective.

So, you must do the technique before the 20 to 30 minute time frame, preferably within the first couple minutes. On a rare occasion, I have been able to stop a migraine that has already progressed pretty far up the curve, but not very often.

Once in a while, the time frame between the first signs of the migraine and "the point of no return" may be longer than the typical 20 to 30 minutes, and extend to an hour or two. When that is the case, then the mindfulness practice will work within that 2- to 3-hour period. However, most of the time, the point of no return occurs closer to the 30 minutes. You probably have a good understanding of your cycle, so judge accordingly.

SIX

Mindfulness Over Migraines
Core Technique

Our first response to pain is to resist it or fight it. This is a natural and normal response triggered by instinct and the survival part of our brain. So, you must first become aware of your resistance to release its power over you.

Although it seems that focusing on the pain you are experiencing would actually increase the pain, the exact opposite is true. This is not the same as being preoccupied with pain or ruminating. We're talking about accepting, embracing and becoming one with your pain. Allowing it to exist in its entirety, which allows it to release.

It is by completely experiencing and embracing our discomfort that we rise above it and live a less painful life. You begin by simply becoming aware of your pain and then exploring it; taking a look at it from the inside and feeling it completely.

Be sure you have read the "Breathing Fundamentals" and "When to do Mindfulness for Migraines" chapters before proceeding, as both of these steps are crucial for the success of the core technique. As discussed previously, the correct method of breathing and timing of your technique is absolutely essential. It must be put into practice shortly after the first signs of a migraine—the sooner the better.

1. Sit or lie down and get comfortable.

   I prefer to lie down, and feel it is more effective this way. However, when that isn't possible, then sitting wherever you are will work. It can be done in your lounger, your office chair or leaning against the wall if you must. You can even pull off the side of the road or into a rest area if you are driving.

2. Close your eyes.

3. Take a deep breath in through the nose and out through the nose. Be sure to breathe from the abdomen, as you learned in

the "Breathing Fundamentals" chapter. Repeat several times to relax. The act of closing the eyes and breathing deeply begins to activate the alpha brainwaves immediately and incite relaxation.

4. With your mind's eye, locate the area where your pain resides. Go inside yourself and zero in precisely on where the pain dwells. Think of yourself as a curious and unbiased scientist on an expedition.

    Where is your pain? Behind your eye, in the middle of your brain, at the top of your head or behind your ear, etc.? Outline the pain with your mind's eye.

    What does your pain look like? Is it square, rectangle, round, spread out, scattered, skinny, narrow, wide, rugged, smooth, sharp, etc.?

    What does your pain feel like? Is it pounding, throbbing, aching, stabbing, pulsating, pinching, burning, etc.? Is it shallow, deep or diffuse? Is it stationary or does it travel?

    Don't use judgmental words like horrific, terrible or awful. You don't want to label or judge the pain, or this will cause the brain to react to it as stress and increase your symptoms. You neutralize the pain by remaining neutral. Venting about how horrible your pain is can be a helpful coping strategy, and there is nothing wrong with that in the right time and place. However, it is best practiced outside this technique. For the sole purpose of this technique, we want to refrain from judgment of the pain.

The pain isn't bad or good; it just is.

Some people like to do a lot of describing, but I don't usually find too much is necessary. You can use as much as you feel is needed to help you locate and connect with the pain. I put the most focus on repeatedly outlining it with my mind's eye.

5.   Explore it; examine it.

Bring your full attention to the spot where it resides. Outline it again with your mind's eye, as many times as needed to really connect with it.

6.   Now, instead of using the breath as the focal point of your meditation as you learned earlier in the "Understanding the Basics of Mindfulness Meditation" chapter, use the pain or discomfort itself as the focal point.

Become aware of nothing but your pain.

Be "with" your pain; don't resist it, don't fight it and don't try to distract yourself.

Go right in there where the pain is and allow it to exist.

Focus on it and sit with it.

Feel it completely.

Just allow it to exist in its entirety without judgment.

Feel it and embrace it completely.

Become "one" with your pain. As if you and your pain are not separate entities.

7. Next, take a deep breath in through the nostrils and, when you breathe out through the nostrils, imagine that you are guiding and pushing the breath into and then out of the area where the pain exists.

    Remember to breathe from your abdomen, not your chest, as you learned in chapter three. Guide the breath on exhale into the area where your pain exists and out through the area where the pain exists.

    Again, take another deep breath in through the nostrils and, when you breathe out through the nostrils, imagine that you are guiding and pushing the breath into and out of the area where the pain exists.

You want to imagine that you are pushing the breath into and then out of the body, in the area where the pain resides. It is the pushing of the breath that moves the pain out. It's as if the breath flows through the pain and then out of the body; and, when it flows out, it carries the pain with it.

Repeat this step several times.

At this point, you should notice that the pain is beginning to dissipate.

8. Now, just be still and bring your full attention to the area of pain again without the breath. Outline it with your mind's eye. Just sit with it quietly.

    Alternatively, you can continue focusing on the pain and breathing deeply until you begin to feel the pain melt away more; and that is exactly what it feels like, a melting or dissolving.

Sometimes the pain literally dissolves in seconds. Sometimes it takes 5, 10, 15 or 30 minutes. On occasion, I have had to engage in the practice for an hour if I have waited too long to do the practice or if it is a particularly powerful trigger. However, most of the time, if it's going to work, it works within the 30 minutes. I am able to alleviate most of my migraines within 15 minutes and sometimes within a couple minutes if I start the practice within a minute or two of the first warning signs.

As you probably know, migraines vary in intensity. Some triggers may produce a very mild migraine, while others are quite severe. The intensity of the migraine will impact how long you must engage in the mindfulness practice, with the most severe requiring more time.

Some migraines may try to come back at a later time, like several hours later. This happens to me occasionally. When that is the case, then just do your mindfulness exercise again. Some can be very stubborn and try to resurface numerous times throughout the day. There are days when I'm doing my mindfulness over migraines technique three or four times a day. I know that this sounds like a lot to go through to relieve pain, but I find it is a much better option than howling and whimpering like a wounded animal for 16 hours. I think you will, too.

Sometimes, I am not able to eliminate the migraine completely, but I can reduce the severity and duration of the migraine. This can be helpful as well because it reduces it enough that I can still function to some degree and I don't have to be confined to the bed.

When You're Too Late

As discussed previously, you must do the practice at the very first sign of an impending migraine. If you're too late or you have one that comes sweeping in too quickly to address, the practice can be used to get through the migraine a little easier.

Prior to my viewing the webinar by Dr. Charles Gant that I mentioned earlier, I was using all the steps I presented above to deal with my migraines and chronic pain except the precise locating and description, and I had not yet discovered the importance of timing. What I had been doing helped me get through the migraine for many years, but did not alleviate it. However, after that webinar, I added locating the precise area of the pain and describing it. It was this zeroing in that enabled me to alleviate the pain more effectively. Then, it was with trial and error that I discovered how crucial the timing is for optimizing the amount of relief that can be achieved.

So, if you're already beyond "the point of no return," you can still use this technique to ease the pain. At this point, it doesn't derail the migraine, but it decreases its intensity, calms down your autonomic nervous system and allows you to go to sleep.

Myofacial Pain

For myself and some others, myofacial pain accompanies migraines quite frequently. This may or may not be the case for you. If it is, then when you're outlining your pain, be sure to locate the pain in the myofacial area as well. The technique works just as beautifully here. Sometimes myofacial pain occurs without a migraine, and relief from myofacial pain alone can always be achieved with the mindfulness technique, usually within a couples minutes. Just do it exactly the same way you would for a migraine.

Other Chronic Pain

Once you know how to apply these principles to alleviating your migraines, it can be applied to pain of all types, even emotional pain. There aren't many things in life more painful than a migraine. In my opinion, it is more painful than childbirth and, in the end, we have no beautiful bundle of joy to make it worth the while. So, if mindfulness can eliminate this type of intense pain, it can work on any pain.

Over the years, I have used this practice successfully for TMJ, IBS, fibromyalgia, myofacial pain, atypical trigeminal neuralgia, grieving the loss of a relationship, grieving in general, backache, gallbladder pain and others. As we discussed earlier, many studies have found that mindfulness is beneficial for chronic pain conditions of all kinds, so there is no limit to the types of pain that you can apply my technique to and find some relief.

Emotional Pain

The same principles can be applied to emotional pain. Instead of physical pain, use the emotional pain as the focal point of the meditation. Feel the full force of the emotion; own it and become one with it. Allow it to exist. Don't judge it or medicate it. This can be used with emotional pain in the current moment or trauma from the past, even trauma that results in post-traumatic stress disorder (PTSD). We can't let go of undesirable or uncomfortable feelings like anger, frustration, sadness, loss, etc., unless we first feel and experience them completely. It is by fully experiencing and embracing our emotions that we live a richer, fuller and more meaningful life.

All Chronic Health Conditions

Although mindfulness is found to be exceptionally beneficial for certain health conditions like migraines, chronic pain, adrenal fatigue, anxiety, depression, heart disease, high blood pressure, dysautonomia, chemical sensitivity and insomnia, there isn't any health condition that cannot benefit from the practice.

Chronic stress is a primary cause or exacerbating factor in all chronic medical and psychiatric disorders because it breaks the body down. Since a primary benefit of mindfulness is reduction of stress, all chronic health conditions respond favorably with a reduction in symptoms.

The driving force of chronic stress is autonomic nervous system dysfunction; the body stays in a state of fight or flight on a frequent basis. Mindfulness directly reduces norepinephrine, the neurotransmitter involved in this process, by turning off the sympathetic nervous system and restoring us to the preferred and regenerative parasympathetic state. This results in immediate relaxation and reduction of stress, and the cascade of positive benefits that follow.

Other Benefits of Mindfulness Meditation

As I mentioned previously, mindfulness has a long list of benefits in addition to relieving migraines or other chronic pain syndromes that will enrich your life.

Stress Management

As we've discussed a variety of times throughout this book, mindfulness has a direct effect on our autonomic nervous system; thus, turning off our sympathetic nervous system and turning on our parasympathetic nervous system. This, of course, results in reduction of stress. Therefore, this makes mindfulness one of the best stress-management techniques you can find—you'll feel more relaxed, and you'll cope more comfortably and effectively with the unavoidable stressors in your life.

Spirituality and Inner Peace

In my definition of spirituality, the components we are trying to achieve include inner peace, contentedness with life, more meaning, depth and purpose in life, connectedness to self and the Universe, living more authentically, developing more empathy and compassion, deeper self-awareness, and a higher level of consciousness. Our spiritual health is largely dependent on how neurotransmitters and the autonomic nervous system are functioning.

Once again, the ability of mindfulness to improve neurotransmitter production and function, and restore balance to the autonomic nervous system, enables us to greatly increase all the components of spirituality, including quieting the mind. The frontal lobes of the brain, which are stimulated with mindfulness meditation, are linked to empathy, compassion and concern for something bigger than self.

In *Breathing: The Master Key to Self Healing*, Dr. Weil tells us that when we focus on our breathing, we are focusing on the non-physical essence (spiritual) of who we are. Essentially, we are connecting with our spiritual self.

Mindfulness also helps us stay grounded in the present moment, quiet the inner commentator, and enhances the quality of life and our overall sense of well-being.

Although our goal when using mindfulness to alleviate migraine headaches or chronic pain of any kind is not for spiritual health, it is impossible not to reap these benefits—they are an inherent component of the practice. We could say that they are a positive side effect.

Creativity, Intuition and Insight

Mindfulness stimulates the areas of the brain and neurotransmitters that generate creativity, intuition and insight. Creative thoughts and ideas begin to flow like a stream. I have so many creative ideas from practicing my mindfulness and deep breathing exercises that I am constantly running for a piece of paper to jot them down, and I am exceptionally insightful and intuitive. The more you practice it, the more creative, insightful and intuitive you become.

Better Relationships

When you are more mindful in your relationships, they are deeper, more meaningful and satisfying. The people in your life feel more appreciated, important and valued, which promotes more harmonious and happier connections. It becomes exceptionally powerful if both people in the relationship practice meditation.

Insomnia and Disrupted Sleep

Studies have found mindfulness to be of significant help with insomnia and disrupted sleep patterns. The direct effect it has on neurotransmitters and the autonomic nervous system provides the body and brain with the ability to turn off the sympathetic nervous system and relax, eliminating the primary cause of sleep problems.

Additionally, both deep breathing and mindfulness stimulate melatonin, our primary hormone that helps us sleep.[1] I use mindfulness and deep breathing every night when I go to bed, and it puts me to sleep in minutes. I often fall asleep during the day if I lie down to do my mindfulness. This makes mindfulness meditation one of the best natural sleep aids you can find.

Improved Mental Health

Because depleted or disrupted neurotransmitters in the brain and autonomic nervous system dysfunction are the root of anxiety, depression, addiction and all other mental health disorders—and one of the primary benefits of mindfulness meditation is that it helps balance these neurotransmitters and the autonomic nervous system—improved mental health is another positive side effect that you will reap from the regular practice of mindfulness. Even if depression, anxiety or other mental health conditions are not an issue for you, you will find that your level of joy, happiness and balance will increase. You'll feel more grounded and connected.

SEVEN

Optimizing Your Mindfulness Over Migraines Benefits

Using mindfulness to eliminate migraines, or chronic pain of any kind, is a skill to be developed; and, just like any other skill, you get better at it with practice. It gets easier and more effective the more often you put it to use.

In time, you'll find that the duration needed to achieve the desired result decreases, and the results will be more impressive. Even with all the years I've been using mindfulness to some degree or another, I continually discover more depth and achieve better results.

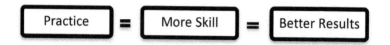

The more you practice mindfulness, the more the frontal lobes of the brain are activated. The more the frontal lobes are activated, the more the locus ceruleus, amygdala and other old brain structures involved in the fight or flight system are diminished. The more diminished the fight or flight, the fewer symptoms experienced. There is a decrease in anxiety, pain, anger, fight, fear and depression, and an increase in relaxation, empathy, compassion, joy and comfort.

However, it's important to be aware that mindfulness is most effective when it is part of a comprehensive and holistic plan to optimize your health. The benefits will be most abundant when it is used in conjunction with a healthy diet plan like the Paleolithic diet, avoidance of environmental toxins with a green lifestyle and nutritional supplements, because a poor diet, nutritional deficiencies and environmental toxins all impair neurotransmitters and functioning of the mind, as well as the autonomic nervous system.

If your brain isn't healthy, and your autonomic nervous system is consistently being challenged with poor diet and environmental toxins, then being mindful can be difficult to achieve. Although mindfulness promotes a healthy brain, it has little to work with if it's nutrient deficient and flooded with toxins. The three together (mindfulness, diet and clean environment) support one another and enhance the effectiveness of each other.

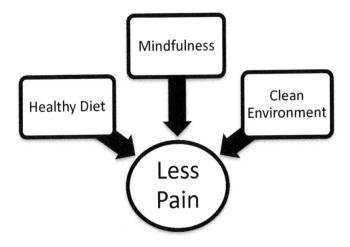

For example, if you're eating sugar, white flour and other junk food, and/or being exposed to chemicals like pesticides and herbicides on a daily basis—all of which disrupt the autonomic nervous system and thrusts you into fight or flight mode—then you're fighting an uphill battle with your mindfulness.

The disruptions that these substances cause to the neurotransmitters in the brain and the autonomic nervous system inhibit or, at the very least, minimize the benefits you can achieve. On the other hand, if you remove those unhealthy foods from your diet and practice green living principles, then you optimize the results you can see.

The Paleolithic diet consists of grass-fed, free-range, organic meat; eggs and wild Alaskan fish; low-starch vegetables; nuts, seeds and low-sugar fruit. Anthropological research tells us that this is the diet that all human beings are genetically programmed to eat, and provides your brain and body the nutrients it needs to function most optimally.[1] I urge you to learn more about it and the benefits it provides. At the very least, you should be eating a diet that consists of real foods in their whole and natural state.

Additionally, the frontal lobes of the brain will also not work adequately if they are not receiving the proper nutrients needed for production, function and transmission. Neurotransmitters and hormones cannot be formed or function properly if the body is missing crucial nutrients like amino acids, fatty acids, B vitamins and minerals, etc. The more deficient you are in nutrients, the more dominant the sympathetic nervous system is likely to become. Undiagnosed nutritional deficiencies or imbalances are abundant in the general population. Assessment for the presence of nutritional deficiencies should be pursued by anyone with migraines.

It's important to note that mindfulness meditation is not a cure-all for migraines; it relieves the pain, but does not cure migraines. By this, I mean that it doesn't stop migraines from returning in the future; but, it will work each and every time they appear to alleviate the pain and improve quality of life. On the other hand, some people report with the regular use of mindfulness, their migraine frequency and intensity decreases.

Mindfulness meditation should not be used as a replacement for other steps in the recovery process like eating healthy, exercise, green living, detoxification, etc., but it should be used in conjunction with these strategies.

Although the autonomic nervous system may be at the core of migraines, dysfunction of the autonomic nervous system is caused by many other contributing factors. If you can identify the underlying triggers that apply to your situation, which are commonly referred to as migraine triggers, then you can reduce the amount of migraines that you experience or possibly eliminate them all together, which is always preferred over managing them or derailing them. Therefore, it's also equally important to identify your primary migraine triggers.

The primary triggers of migraines that can result in autonomic nervous system dysfunction that you should investigate include:

- Omega 3 fatty acid deficiency
- magnesium deficiency
- B vitamin deficiencies
- cavitations
- trauma to the trigeminal nerve
- food sensitivities

- other nutritional deficiencies
- neurotransmitter depletion
- candida overgrowth
- hormone imbalance
- parasites or bacterial overgrowth
- heavy metal toxicity
- TMJ
- structural misalignment
- hypoglycemia
- pesticide exposure or other common everyday chemicals

If you'd like to learn more about how to identify if these factors apply to your situation, contact me for a phone consultation, or look for a practitioner in your area that practices functional medicine or environmental medicine.

The greatest thing about mindfulness meditation is that it will not only alleviate your migraine headaches, it will also assist you in the process of recovery for any of these other underlying causes and conditions, reduce stress, and promote more inner peace along the way.

The aspect that I love the most about mindfulness is that it is a practice that merges the worlds of science and spirituality. It's a strategy to improve mental and physical health, and a spiritual practice all wrapped into one.

Additionally, since it costs you absolutely nothing and be can be performed in the comfort of your own home, or anywhere else you might be, it's one of the most affordable, practical and natural self-care strategies to be found—providing us with an abundant sense of empowerment.

Because of its impact on immune function, the autonomic nervous system, the brain and neurotransmitters, mindfulness will benefit your life in ways that go far beyond pain relief. It enhances our physical, emotional and spiritual health simultaneously by stimulating those neurotransmitters that decrease stress, improve mood, heighten our sense of well-being in the world, and helps us achieve higher states of consciousness, creativity and awareness. It is truly one of the most supreme holistic techniques available to optimize your physical, emotional and spiritual health overall.

In its simplest form, mindfulness is a technique to achieve better health and spiritual development; however, it is much more than that. As it is practiced more frequently, it becomes integrated into a way of living that enriches your day-to-day life. Your life essentially becomes a type of meditation.

The miracle of mindfulness is that it minimizes the experiences we typically consider negative that cause suffering (pain, depression, grief, sadness, trauma, stress, anxiety, etc.) but, at the same time, it enhances the experiences we typically consider pleasurable (joy, happiness, inner peace and serenity), simultaneously—providing us with a more meaningful and richer life.

Not only that, it is completely free, requires no visit to a health practitioner's office, fits within any belief system and is available at your fingertips 24-hours a day. This makes mindfulness a cost-effective approach that is within reach for everyone, even those with the most challenging financial conditions.

Now, you can take these principles and apply them to all your life experiences. Mindfulness can be practiced in every area of your life that you can think of: making love, spending time with nature, taking a walk, cleaning the house, working, writing, gardening, watching a movie, washing the dishes, listening to music, breathing, drinking water, engaging in conversation, etc. Virtually everything and anything you do can be done in a more mindful manner.

By being fully present and aware of each experience—even the pain and discomfort, or simply quieting our inner dialogue—we live a deeper, richer and more fulfilling life, and optimize our health physically, emotionally and spiritually at the same time. There is no other technique, procedure, treatment or remedy on the planet that can match these benefits, so I encourage you to take full advantage of what mindfulness has to offer.

Notes

The following is an overview of all the sources cited within this book. You will find the full details of all cited references, as well as other recommended reading, in the bibliography.

Chapter One

1. Gant, Mindfulness Webinar
2. Kabat-Zinn and others. "The Clinical Use of Mindfulness Meditation for Self-Regulation of Chronic Pain"
3. Kabat-Zinn, "Four Year Follow-Up of a Meditation-Based Program"
4. Gaylord, "Mindfulness vs. Support Groups for Irritable Bowel Syndrome"
5. Wachholtz and Pargament, "Migraines & Meditation"

6. Zeidan and others, "Brain Mechanisms Supporting the Modulation of Pain by Mindfulness Meditation"

7. Wildmind, "What is Mindfulness?"

Chapter Two

1. Clarity Seminars, "Effects of Stress on Health and Productivity"

2. 4 Mind 4 Life: Good Health Tips, http://4mind4life.com/blog/

3. Gant, Endocrine Stress Webinar; Weil, *Breathing*

Chapter Four

1. Gant, Mindfulness Webinar

2. Kabat-Zinn, http://www.umassmed.edu/content.aspx?id=41252

Chapter Six

1. Wong, "Melatonin and Meditation"

Chapter Seven

1. Cordain, *The Paleo Diet*; Sears, "Missing Link Ate Meat"

Bibliography

The works listed here are a starting point for those interested in more information about topics covered in this book. The list includes all works cited in the text as well as recommended reading. All websites listed were last accessed in June 2012.

Carlson, L. E. and S.N. Garland. "Impact of Mindfulness-Based Stress Reduction (MBSR) on Sleep, Mood, Stress and Fatigue Symptoms in Cancer Outpatients." *International Journal of Behavioral Medicine*, 12(4), (2005): 278–85.

Clarity Seminars. "Effects of Stress on Health and Productivity." http://www.clarityseminars.com/stress_clinical_research.html *Clinical Psychiatry*, 62 (2), (2006).

Cordain, Loren. *The Paleo Diet: Lose Weight and Get Healthy by Eating the Food You Were Designed to Eat.* Wiley, 2002.

Davidson, R., et. al. "Alterations in Brain and Immune Function Produced by Mindfulness Meditation." *Psychosomatic Medicine*, 65 (2003): 564–570.

4 Mind 4 Life: Mental Health Tips. http://4mind4life.com/blog/

Gant, Charles, MD. Mindfulness Webinar. http://www.cegant.com/

———. Endocrine Stress Webinar. http://www.cegant.com/

Gaylord, Susan, PhD. "Mindfulness vs. Supports for Irritable Bowel Syndrome." Presented at University of North Carolina at Chapel Hill during Digestive Disease Week, May 7, 2011.

Ilades, Chris, MD. "Meditation for Headache Relief." Everyday Health. http://www.everydayhealth.com/headache-migraine/headache-relief-meditation.aspx

Kabat-Zinn, Jon, PhD. "Four Year Follow-Up of a Meditation-Based Program." *Clinical Journal of Pain*, 2 (1986).

———. http://www.umassmed.edu/content.aspx?id=41252

Kabat-Zinn, Jon, PhD, et al. "The Clinical Use of Mindfulness Meditation for Self-Regulation of Chronic Pain." *Journal of Behavioral Medicine*, Volume 1 (1978), Volume 35 (2012).

Rosenzweig, S., et al. "Mindfulness-Based Stress Reduction for Chronic Pain Conditions: Variation in Treatment Outcomes and Role of Home Meditation Practice." J Psychosom Res, 2010. 68(1): 29–36.

Sears, Al, MD. "Missing Link Ate Meat." http://www.alsearsmd.com/missing-link-ate-meat/

Wachholtz, Amy, B. and Kenneth I. Pargament. "Migraines & Meditation: Does Spirituality Matter." *Journal of Behavioral Medicine*, 31 (2008):351–366.

Weil, Andrew, MD. *Breathing: The Master Key to Self Healing* (CD). Sounds True Incorporated, 2001.

Wildmind. "What is Mindfulness?" http://www.wildmind.org/applied/daily-life/what-is-mindfulness

Wong, Cathy. "Melatonin and Meditation." About.com. http://altmedicine.about.com/cs/mindbody/a/Melatonin.htm

Zeidan F., et al. "Brain Mechanisms Supporting the Modulation of Pain by Mindfulness Meditation." J Neurosci, 31(14), (2011): 5540–5548.

About the Author

Cynthia Perkins, M.Ed., is an author of more than ten self-help books, a holistic health counselor and sobriety coach who has used mindfulness-based techniques for managing chronic pain syndromes for more than twenty years. She holds a bachelor's degree in psychology and a master's degree in counseling.

Her holistic health services—which focus on optimizing mental, physical and spiritual health with diet, nutrition, green living, mindfulness, deep breathing exercises and lifestyle changes—can be found at Holistic Help: http://www.holistichelp.net/

Cynthia's alcoholism and addiction services can be found by visiting http://www.alternativesforalcoholism.com

Cynthia is also an adult sex educator. Services for this issue can be found at Helping Couples Have Great Sex:
http://www.smolderingembers.com

Other Books and Booklets by Cynthia

Get Sober Stay Sober: The Truth About Alcoholism

Candida Secrets

What Your Psychologist Hasn't Told You About Anxiety & Depression

Living Life to the Fullest: Creative Coping Strategies for Managing Chronic Illness

Quit Smoking with Ease – Naturally

Meditating for Health

How to Break Your Sugar Addiction Today

Mindfulness Over Chronic Pain: Eliminate Your Pain in Minutes . . . Naturally and Affordably

CPSIA information can be obtained
at www.ICGtesting.com
Printed in the USA
LVHW03s1528140618
580752LV00013B/664/P